Spirituality and Nursing

Shirley Brydie, Ph.D., R.N.

VANTAGE PRESS
New York

The opinions and instructions expressed herein are solely those of the author. Each individual should seek the advice of his or her own physician before starting any new medical program.

Cover design by Polly McQuillen

FIRST EDITION

Published by Vantage Press, Inc.
419 Park Ave. South, New York, NY 10016

Manufactured in the United States of America
ISBN: 0-533-14658-5

Library of Congress Catalog Card No.: 2003094076

0 9 8 7 6 5 4 3 2 1

To the man in my life, Arthur Holmes, and my children, John, Suchilla, Jason, my grandson, Elijah from whom the idea of this project was founded, and to Kyla. I thank them all for their patience and tolerance of all the times I could not be at home with them because I needed to be in school. They were a constant source of support and encouragement.

I also thank GOD for giving me the strength and endurance to continue with my full-time job as Nurse Clinician for OB/GYN/ONCOLOGY, organizational and spiritual commitments and the friends that understood my missing various activities.

The idea for this project came about with the birth of my premature grandson. Elijah was born at 27 weeks gestation weighing only two pounds; but because of spiritual, emotional dedication of our family praying for him, applying touch therapies in an effort to promote a caring and healing environment I am proud to say that after three years, Elijah, though he has some delays, is doing well. Noting the power of prayer and spirituality and nursing.

Without God I am nothing

Contents

Preface

Brydie, Shirley (2002):
Spirituality and Nursing

The ambition of this thesis was to explore and understand the nursing process from a holistic or alternative care perspective. Historical exploration included attitudes, preparation and expectations.

The specific aim was to identify the need that patients increasingly are seeking alternative or complementary therapies and demanding the integration of spiritual care into their therapy, nurses are expected to offer a holistic approach to their services. As a result, the nurse becomes responsible for assessing not only the physical but also the spiritual needs of patients. This integration of mind, body, and spirit is referred to as holism. In this way, medical remedies are no longer adequate in restoring a patient's balanced energy state; rather, addressing the spiritual needs via alternative therapies (e.g., praying, touch therapies, story-telling, music, and pastoral care) may encourage a patient's complete recovery.

In summary, this research is to provide a historical perspective of spirituality in nursing to educate and support contemporary nurses in the twenty-first century as they shift from providing traditional to alternative services.

Keywords: Holism, praying, touch therapies, story-telling, music, pastoral care.

Author's Note

Dissertation Proposal

Dissertation Title: Spirituality and Nursing

I. Problem Statement

As patients increasingly are seeking alternative or complementary therapies and demanding the integration of spiritual care into their therapy, nurses are expected to offer a holistic approach to their services. As a result, the nurse becomes responsible for assessing not only the physical but also the spiritual needs of patients. This integration of mind, body, and spirit is referred to as holism. In this way, medical remedies are no longer sufficient in restoring a patient's balanced energy state: rather, addressing the spiritual needs via alternative therapies (e.g., praying, touch therapies, story-telling, music, pastoral care) may encourage a patient's recovery.

The paradigm shift from traditional to alternative nursing practices requires not only organizational, but also educational support. As a result, continuing education addressing issues of spirituality and healing for nurses is essential. Nurses who are properly educated about the implications of not only the patient's, but also their own spirituality, are better equipped to provide patients with holistic healing.

In addition, organizational support, such as the formulation of policies or operating procedures that incorporate spiritually based practices into traditional nursing methods, encourages the spiritual development both of the patient and the caregiver. Moreover, an institution that has implemented a strong, continuous effort to promote conscious spiritual health-care behaviors in its employees is more likely to exhibit a thriving healing culture. Finally, as services provided by nurses shift from traditional to alternative or complementary, the nurse's role will expand to encompass the spiritual in addition to the physical and psychological care of patients.

The purpose of this research is to provide a historical perspective of spirituality in nursing in order to educate and support contemporary nurses of the twenty-first century as they shift from providing traditional to alternative services.

II. Background

Spirituality is a tendency to gain meaning through a sense of relatedness to other dimensions that transcend the self, creating healing of the mind, body, and spirit (O'Brien, 1999; Wardell, 2001; Skokan, 2000). Consequently, spirituality is the basis of holistic approaches to nursing. Current research suggests that patients who engage in spiritual practices (e.g., prayer, touch therapies) have improved outcomes. Nurses' roles shift from providing physical care to ministering to the patient's whole body, mind, and spirit in order to encourage healing.

As if the integration of alternative therapies were not enough, Wong and Pang (2000) assert that health care cultures view holism in vastly diverse ways. With respect to Eastern medicine, the focus of therapy is to restore balance and harmony to the body, specifically the yin and yang. In addition, medical remedies alone prove to be insufficient in restoring a balanced, healthy state. Mendyka (2000) concurs with Wong and Pang (2000) and adds that a patient's illness is a cultural experience that nurses should be cognizant of when addressing the unique physiological, psychosocial, cultural, and spiritual needs of patients.

The medical practices of nurses in ancient civilizations provide foundations for current health-care services. O'Brien (1999) asserts that early Christians opened their homes and ministered to individuals in physical and spiritual need in order to imitate the actions of Jesus Christ. By the fourth, fifth, and sixth centuries, nursing became institutionalized. In the sixteenth, seventeenth, eighteenth, and nineteenth centuries, religious nursing communities experienced moderate to exponential growth. In fact, a few of these orders such as the Daughters of Charity and the Nightingale nursing community, have not only provided significant historical contributions to nursing and healthcare practices but also are still in existence today (O'Brien, 1999). In the twenty-first century, parish nursing is a specialty practice based on early Christian healing ministry, facilitating the holistic health of a community of faith (Brendtro, 2000).

Spiritual care interventions that a nurse may implement in a regimen may include, but are not limited to, touch therapies (e.g., healing touch, Reiki, therapeutic touch), pastoral care, prayer, rituals, story-telling, and music (Dunn, 2000; O'Brien, 19999; Wright, 2000, Skokan, 2000; Ameling, 2000). These interventions may or may not be religiously based. However, their focus is to address the spiritual needs of ill patients and integrate the mind, body, and spirit in a holistic approach to healing.

III. Annotated Bibliography

Ameling A. "Prayer: An ancient healing practice becomes new again." *Holistic Nursing Practice.* 2000; 14 (3) :40–48.

Ameling defines prayer, in general, as well as describing the many forms of prayer. Moreover, the article cites studies in which the healing effects of particular types of prayer were realized.

Brendtro M., Leuning C. "Nurses in churches: A population-focused clinical option." *Journal of Nursing Education.* 2000; 39 (6) :285.

This article describes the history and mission of parish nursing. In addition, Brendtro and Leuning review the specialized education that parish nursing students must encounter.

Dunn K., Horgas A. "The prevalence of prayer as a spiritual self-care modality in elders." *Journal of Holistic Nursing.* 2000; 18 (4) :337–351.

Dunn and Horgas present their study on prayer in elderly patients as a means to cope with illness and/or death. The authors determined that 96% of elderly participants used prayer to cope with stress in their lives.

Mendkya B. "Exploring the culture of nursing: A theory-driven practice." *Holistic Nursing Practice.* 2000; 15 (1) :32–51.

Mendkya reviews Watson's Model of Human Care in an effort to comprehend the culture behind the holistic nursing practice. The author concludes that, as nurses draw upon Watson's Model, they are better equipped to recognize the cultural diversity of patients and offer to them the appropriate holistic therapy.

O'Brien M. "Spirituality in nursing: Standing on holy ground." In: O'Brien, M.Ed. *Spirituality in Nursing: Standing on Holy Ground.* Jones and Bartlett: Boston. 1999 :1–17.

This chapter in O'Brien's book serves as an introduction to the concept of spirituality in nursing. As a jumping off point for the book, this chapter provides definitions upon which the remainder of the book will build and develop.

O'Brien M. "A spiritual history of nursing." In: O'Brien, M.Ed. *Spirituality in Nursing; Standing on Holy Ground.* Jones and Bartlett: Boston. 1999 :21–52.

O'Brien provides a general history of nursing with respect to spirituality starting in the Pre-Christian Era and ending in the Post-Reformation Period. The major emphasis of the chapter is on Christian-based nursing history.

O'Brien M. "Spiritual care: The nurse's role." In: O'Brien, M.Ed. *Spirituality in Nursing: Standing on Holy Ground.* Jones and Bartlett: Boston. 1999 :118–142.

O'Brien touches on the nature of the nurse's role with respect to providing spiritual care to patients and defines it in terms of religious traditions. In addition, O'Brien mentions religious and spiritual interventions that nurses may use to provide patients with the spiritual care they require.

Skokan L., Bader D. "Spirituality and healing." *Health Progress.* 2000; 81 (1) :38.

Skokan and Bader review a study conducted by the Sisters of Providence Health System (PHS) whose purpose was to show that spirituality is an essential dimension of health and well-being. In particular, this

PHS study focuses on the influences of spirituality and spiritual experiences on the health and well-being of chronically ill patients.

Wardell D. "Spirituality and healing touch participants." *Journal of Holistic Nursing.* 2001; 19 (1) :71–86.

Wardell assessed whether there was a difference in the spirituality of nurses and non-nurses trained in healing touch. The author found that individuals with higher levels of training exhibited a heightened sense of spiritual awareness.

Wong T., Pang M. "Holism and caring: Nursing in Chinese health care culture." *Holistic Nursing Practice.* 2000; 15 (1) :12–21.

Wong and Pang examine holism within the historical and cultural context of nursing in the Chinese culture. The authors review the concepts of holism as defined in terms of the Chinese community and attempt to understand the reasons why the Chinese community views nursing in a particular way.

Wright S. "Praying for good health." *Nursing Standard.* 2000; 15 (2) :27.

Wright provides a brief review of the literature that points to the effectiveness of prayer in healing. The author cautions that, although prayer has been shown to affect health and is thus worthy of consideration, improved assessment tools for nurses to identify the spiritual needs of patients are imperative.

IV. Proposed Methodology

A historical literature review of spirituality in nursing will be conducted in order to examine the role of spirituality in healing, holism, and caring for the total patient.

Dissertation

Presented to

Clayton College of Natural Health

In Partial Fulfillment
Of the Requirements for the Degree
Doctor of Natural Health
July 30, 2001

One

Introduction

With the advent of alternative and complementary therapies, nurses have been shouldered with the additional responsibility of integrating spiritual care into their services. As health-care strategies shift from the traditional to holistic, healing of the spirit, as well as the mind and the body, becomes involved when planning a therapeutic regimen. Consequently, nurses are faced with the challenge of assessing and caring for the spiritual, in addition, to the physical needs of the patients.

The purpose of this research is to educate and support nurses in the twenty-first century by gaining a historical perspective of spirituality and nursing. Undoubtedly, nursing has a spiritual basis dating back to the early Christian era when Christians opened their homes to people in physical and spiritual need in order to imitate Jesus Christ. This spiritual element continues throughout the history of nursing and has had a significant resurgence with the onset of alternative and complementary therapies.

Today, nurses can use the historical background provided in this thesis to model their practices, which address the spiritual needs of their patients. Consequently, nurses who are more familiar with the implications of their own spirituality, as well as spirituality in healing, will be better equipped to meet the spiritual needs of their patients.

Nature of Problem

The incorporation of spiritual care into current health-care practices has escalated with the emergence of alternative and complementary therapies. A recent poll cited by O'Brien (1999) indicated that 74 percent of Americans thought that their health-care providers should initiate a discussion of their (the patient's) spiritual beliefs, refer them to a spiritual advisor (e.g., priest, rabbi), or integrate prayer into their treatment regimen. Moreover, 90 percent of patients felt that spirituality should be addressed in end-of-life situations. Approximately 54 percent of patients recommended that health-care professionals learn innovative ways in which to incorporate spirituality into their treatment strategies (O'Brien, 1999).

By looking to the past for clues for integrating spirituality in nursing practices, nurses become better educated and trained to meet the spiritual, as well as the physical, needs of their patients. Spirituality in nursing dates back to pre-Christian societies in which religion was influential in treating the inform and gods were offered libations and gifts in return for health-related favors.

Nurses of early Christian societies modeled their services after those of Jesus Christ and ministered to the community's physical and spiritual needs. Today, we refer to these Christian nurses as parish nurses. Although times have changed, spirituality in nursing consistently implies a belief in a higher authority transcending physical, material needs to integrate the mind and spirit.

Spiritually based therapies address the health of the whole patient by integrating the mind, body, and spirit. For example, touch therapies may involve direct (e.g., healing touch, therapeutic touch, Reiki) or indirect (e.g., supportive greeting) contact with the intention of altering the patient's energy system to promote self-healing. In fact, the integration of touch therapies, in particular, decreases the stress levels and pain medication used for pre- and post-operative patients (Alandydy, 1999).

Like touch therapies, prayer integrates the spiritual side of healing in order to have a positive effect on the physical state of the patient. Dunn and Horgas (2000) reported that elderly participants who engaged in prayer frequently, as an alternative treatment, were more likely to be optimistic and self-reliant in their coping strategies.

Similarly, Wright (2000) cites data from a study that indicates that patients receiving prayer exhibited significant health improvement and have fewer medical interventions and complications. Moreover, the National Center for Complementary and Alternative Medicine (NCCAM) identifies prayer as a significant treatment option in the category of mind and body control (Dunn, 2000). Arguably, spiritual interventions, such as prayer and touch therapies, empower the patient and are instrumental for the patient to maintain his or her health and well-being.

Although spiritually based holistic approaches to nursing are being reintroduced, some practitioners are reluctant to incorporate this into the patient's therapy. First, the nurse may be uncomfortable with his/her own spirituality or with engaging a patient in an exchange on religious topics. Secondly, nurses do not have adequate

3

models from which to draw upon experience and model their behavior. In providing nurses with adequate training in spiritual practices as well as adequate organizational support to integrate spirituality and holism into their services, nurses will be helped to meet the spiritual needs of patients.

Definition of Terms

SPIRITUALITY: The tendency to acquire meaning through a sense of relatedness to a higher authority in order to promote the healing of the mind, body, and spirit. Spirituality may or may not involve organized religion.

HOLISM: A system that promotes the intimate connection of body, mind, and spirit in treating the whole patient.

TOUCH THERAPIES: Energy-based therapies that involve direct or indirect touching in an effort to heal the body's damaged energy system. Touch therapies are based on the idea that the illness is a symptom of an imbalanced energy system; therefore, touch therapy practitioners assess the patient's energy imbalances and transfer energy from themselves to the patient in order to restore balance. These therapies include therapeutic touch (TT), healing touch (HT), and Reiki.

PRAYER: A request or petition to a higher power for a favorable outcome. Prayer may be active or passive, as either the patient or additional supportive people may engage in prayer on one's behalf.

PARISH NURSE: A registered nurse who provides holistic health care services to a faith community. They function as organizers, educators, and liaisons between the faith and health-care communities in an effort to encourage the relationship between one's faith and health.

PASTORAL CARE: Interventions performed by religious ministers to address the spiritual and religious needs of patients.

SPIRITUAL WELL-BEING: An affirmation of life in a relationship (e.g., nurse-patient) to encourage a patient's wholeness with God, self, community, and the environment. Spiritual well-being results from a patient's healthy spirituality and serves as a basis for holistic nursing care.

HEALING: The process of achieving a state of spiritual well-being, peace, and joy, free from abnormal anxiety, guilt, and feeling of sinfulness. It is not necessarily treating a patient for a condition.

Two
Literature Review

Introduction

Nursing is a sacred ministry of health care or health promotion to patients both sick and well, who need caregiving, support, or education to aid them in achieving, regaining, or maintaining a state of wholeness, including wellness of body, mind, and spirit.

—O'Brien (1999)

Spirituality in nursing involves the belief in a higher authority and the human traits of honesty, love, caring, and compassion, which transcend from the material to the mystical realm, creating healing of the body, mind, and spirit. Spirituality may or may not involve organized religion (O'Brien, 1999). Wardell (2001) and Skokan and Bader (2000) define spirituality as the tendency to acquire meaning through a sense of relatedness to dimensions that transcend the self in such a way that it empowers rather than devalues an individual. Moreover, spirituality is a life affirmation, which nurtures wholeness, as individuals strive to live their lives according to their own values (Wardell, 2001).

Spirituality is the basis of holistic approaches to nursing. In this way, the nurse ministers to the patient's entire body, mind, and spirit to encourage a state of wholeness or wellness throughout the body (O'Brien, 1999). Despite the advances in evidence-based research, O'Callaghan (2001) adds that there are still instances in which nurses work in environments where ritual and tradition supersede basic research evidence. Patients increasingly are demanding that health-care professionals incorporate spiritual care into their practices. In fact, 74 percent of Americans suggest that health-care providers lead a discussion of a patient's spiritual beliefs, refer them to a spiritual advisor (e.g., priest, rabbi), or institute prayer as part of the patient's treatment. In addition, 90 percent of patients indicated that they desired spirituality to be addresses in end-of-life situations. As many as 54 percent of patients indicated that healthcare professionals need to learn ways in which to incorporate spirituality into healthcare (O'Brien, 1999). As patients seek alternative or complementary therapies, nurses increasingly are asked to integrate a holistic approach to their care regimen (Koehn, 2000).

Prior to incorporating spirituality into health-care practices, it is essential that nurses identify their own spirituality and personal belief system prior to administering holistic approaches to therapy for patients. Whether or not nurses are comfortable with supplying patients with spiritual care is always a consideration; however, it is the nurse's responsibility to assess the spiritual needs of the patient and refer them to the appropriate pastoral services (O'Brien, 1999).

Nursing and Holism

Holistic nursing promotes the intimate connection of body, mind, spirit. According to Wong and Pang (2000), the World Health Organization (WHO) defines health as a state of physical, social, psychological, and spiritual well-being. Slater, Maloney, Krau and Eckert (1999) investigate the process of integrating holism into nursing practice. Based on data collected via interviews (n = 18), Slater et al. found that eight concepts consistently emerged: 1) the pathway through which the nurses recognized that they were not conforming to mainstream nursing practices, 2) support from others in their efforts, 3) nurses striving for balance, 4) increase in emphasis on self-care, 5) an alternative understanding of consciousness, 6) their personal presence in nursing practices, 7) an increased spiritual awareness, and 8) recognition of human energy fields as sources of health. Consequently, nurses recognized that holistic approaches improved self-care and life-style parameter to address the body, mind, and emotional and spiritual states to consciously assist in healing. Such healing can be facilitated via meditation or communion with a divine being (Slater, 1999).

In recognizing and deepening their own spirituality, nurses were better equipped to address the spiritual needs of patients. Nurses in Slater et al.'s study (1999) achieved physical, emotional, mental, and spiritual balance via personal lifestyle of work, play, nutrition, rest, alternate self-healing efforts, and spiritual practices. Nurses who developed a more balanced life, were increasingly aware of their own presence as a primary tool for healing. Slater et al. designated presence as the hallmark of a holistic nurse as he/she is available to patients allowing them time and space to heal. Presence may be provided to patients via physical, mental, emotional, and spiritual tactics, in addition to surrounding the patient with healing energy. As nurses develop their own spirituality and self-awareness, they enter into their journey of becoming holistic nurses (Slater, 1999). As health-care corporations adopt a behavior, language, and communication, patient care is depersonalized. As a result, patients experience conflicts with the goals of the new health-care system and their own perception of human service that touches their hopes, fears, and emotions. In response to this, Agnew (1999) asserts that Catholic systems such as the Daughters of Charity (St. Louis, MO) have created programs such as Spirit Care, which moves beyond the goals of curing the patient and strives to promote spirituality and healing.

The focus of Spirit Care is to provide remedies for spiritual disease, such as the patient's lack of hope, purpose, and meaning by encouraging the patients to repair lost connections to his/her family and community. In order to train adequately nurses affiliated with Spirit Care, the system provides caregivers with videos to aid them in identifying and addressing spiritual health care issues on a day-to-day basis. In order to design an adequate spiritual care program, Agnew (1999) suggests that an organization develop a plan of action that is based on respect for the patient as well as the identification of outcomes to track the progress of spiritual healing.

Holism and Cultural Diversity

The ways in which different health-care cultures conceptualize holism and caring may be vastly diverse. Specifically, Wong and Pang (2000) analyze the concepts of

9

holism and caring within the Chinese culture and ground it in a historical context. The focus of Eastern medicine is to counteract imbalances in the body that are considered the sources of illness. In order to restore balance and harmony to the body, Chinese medical therapies, such as herbal medicine, massage therapy, moxibustion, and acupuncture, are used to encourage the natural tendency of the body to restore balanced state. In this way, medical therapies aim at restoring balance to the two archetypal poles of yin and yang (Wong, 2000).

According to Wong and Pang, the medical remedies themselves are not adequate in restoring a patient's balanced state; rather, the ways in which the patient is cared for and their relationship to the therapeutic environment is important in restoring harmony. Traditionally, Chinese family members accept the moral obligation to care for their sick relatives. Consequently, Chinese nurses are seen as outsiders to this private sphere and are undervalued in Chinese society today. Wong and Pang (2000) conclude that, as a result of the lack of cultural understanding, Chinese individuals view professional nursing with ambivalence. Studies such as Wong and Pang's provide clues detailing the nature of nursing within different cultures, as well as the ways in which nurses contribute to people's health and well-being (Wong, 2000).

Similarly, Mendyka (2000) identifies culture as an imperative component for providing holistic care in nursing. Mendyka cites Watson's Model for Human Care in order to exemplify how human illness becomes a cultural event and how nursing is an interpersonal or intersubjective process. Moreover, comprehending the patient's cultural experience of illness is instrumental in complementing the nurse-patient relationship in the holistic nursing practice.

A contradiction to holistic care arises when nurses tend to adopt cultural models or explanations of illness that essentialize the illness, reducing it to human "parts" as opposed to the "whole." In this way, patient conditions are reduced to technical issues that ignore human uniqueness or cultural diversity.

Mendyka concludes that Watson's Model of Human Care serves as a blueprint to aid health care providers in offering more culturally appropriate and meaningful health care for patients and their families. In this way, patients are seen as vital beings with unique physiological, psychological, cultural, and spiritual dimensions. In recognizing this, nurses can provide more culturally sensitive care to patients in order to have a positive impact on the health status of the patient (Mendyka, 2000).

With respect to the culture of aging, Holstein (2000) suggests that, by incorporating various religious views, nurses can adopt a world view that transforms their public and private relationships with elders. In this way, the culture of ageism as understood by nurses and family members has an enormous impact on how individuals experience old age. In some religiously dominated cultures, elders serve a valuable role in developing the cultural, political, and economic priorities of the community. Conversely, as elders are not integrated into society, their dignity and integrity are compromised. Holstein concludes that, from a religious perspective, God is honored by honoring and tending to the needs of the elderly who represent the presence of the spirit (Holstein, 2000). In effect, this aged culture can share a deeper perspective with caregivers that may provide clues into spirituality.

11

Historical Background

As nursing practices enter the twenty-first century, nurses draw upon the vision, created by the spirituality of pioneer nurses to inform, strengthen, and support their contemporary caregiving (O'Brien, 1999). The profession of nursing is rooted in a women's natural role of caring for sick relatives and community members (Marshall, 1999).

Pre-Christian Period

The medical practices of ancient civilizations provide foundations for the health-care practices of Christian nurses. Four civilizations that have greatly influenced the art and science of modern medicine are Egypt, Greece, Rome, and Israel. Usually, individuals who provided nursing care in pre-Christian societies were slaves. In all of these pre-Christian societies, religion was influential in nursing the sick. In some cases, gods were offered libations and gifts in petition for favors related to health and illness (O'Brien, 1999).

Christianity and Nursing

Early Christian societies viewed nursing the infirm or injured as an honor, and those individuals who provided nursing care were well respected. O'Brien (1999) indicates that early Christians ministered to those in physical and spiritual need in an effort to imitate the actions of Jesus Christ. As a result, early Christians, such as deacons and deaconesses, were eager to open their homes and hearts to those who required physical and emotional care. In the third and fourth centuries, Roman matrons were women who used their power and wealth to support the charitable work of attending to the sick by founding hospitals and convents. Deacons and deaconesses, as well as Roman matrons, served as the harbingers of professional nursing in the Christian church (O'Brien, 1999). With the creation of monasteries in the fourth, fifth, and sixth centuries, nursing became institutionalized. As a result, Christian men and women became cloistered and were committed to nursing the sick in the community. Despite the fact that monasteries created a formalized nursing care program for the physically ill, their services neglected to address the needs of those patients suffering from mental illness or other cognitive impairments (O'Brien, 1999).

Post-Reformation Nursing

By the sixteenth century, more than a hundred female, religious nursing orders had been created for the sole purpose of providing nursing care to the infirm. Moderate growth of nursing communities continued during the seventeenth, eighteenth, and nineteenth centuries. While some orders have survived throughout history to care for the ill and infirm, others, which were short-lived, provided little historical significance.

O'Brien (1999) focuses on Catholic and Protestant orders that provided significant historical contributions to nursing and health-care practices and are in existence today. The Daughters of Charity of St. Vincent de Paul adhere to the spirit and spirituality of St. Vincent de Paul. The Nightingale nursing community, led by Florence

Nightingale, were spiritually motivated to minister to the sick in the Crimean War. Both of these communities continue to serve the sick poor in contemporary society in both the United States and abroad (O'Brien, 1999).

Touch Therapies

As nursing moves toward integrative health-care in an effort to promote a caring and healing environment, touch or energy-based therapies are implemented as part of the plan. According to O'Brien (1999), loving, empathetic, compassionate touch is an essential element in the nursing theology of caring. Physical touch includes the laying of hands, holding a patient's hand, or stroking their forehead; however, verbal touching refers to offering words of comfort and support or a cheerful greeting (O'Brien, 1999). In addition, energy-based therapies include Therapeutic Touch (TT), acupressure, shiatsu, and Healing Touch (HT) (Wardell, 2001).

HT, in particular, implements physical touch to influence or heal the human energy system. In this way, HT attempts to restore and maintain balance within a patient's energy field. Consequently, alterations in the human energy system impact a patient's physical, emotional, mental, and spiritual health. Increased spiritual awareness is one of the outcomes of both practicing and receiving HT (Wardell, 2001).

The spiritual awareness of personnel performing HT therapy may have an impact on patient outcomes. Wardell (2001) assessed nurses and non-nurses (n = 477) who perform HT to determine if a difference exists in their perception of spirituality. In this way, the author proposes that nurses who complete higher training levels

14

have a greater spiritual awareness. The curriculum, which serves as higher education for HT practitioners, has four levels ending in HT certification. The spirituality of practitioners was assessed using instruments such as the Spiritual Perspective Scale and the Questionnaire on Spiritual and Religious Attitudes (QSRA). Wardell found that spirituality in nurses and non-nurses did not differ significantly.

However, there was a significant difference in the spiritual perspective of individuals with respect to the level of training in HT. As a result, Wardell confirmed that those individuals who are products of higher levels of the educational program had a heightened sense of spiritual awareness. Aside from potentially exerting a positive impact on patient outcomes, Wardell concludes that HT meets both the spiritual needs of the practitioner and the client (Wardell, 2001).

Similarly, therapeutic touch (TT) is a meditative healing technique that implements physical contact (e.g., laying of hands), non-contact interventions (e.g., voice, eye contact), or a combination of both in order to modulate the body's energy fields (Hayes, 1999; Straneva, 2000). According to Ramnarine-Singh (1999), a TT practitioner passes his/her hands two to six inches above the patient's body from head to feet and detects subtle energy cues that may indicate an imbalance. Based on these energy cues, the TT practitioner plans a treatment strategy to direct energy to the patient's depleted areas (Ramnarine-Singh, 1999).

Anecdotal reports document the restorative properties of TT as it transfers energy from the practitioner to the patients to promote self-healing. For example, Straneva cites a study that assesses the physical benefits of the laying of hands in a population of ill individuals.

15

The physical effects of TT were investigated by drawing baseline and post-treatment blood samples to test the hemoglobin. Hemoglobin was chosen because it is the most sensitive measure of oxygen absorption. Data indicate that those patients receiving TT had significantly greater hemoglobin levels, which was consistent with later studies (Straneva, 2000).

Spiritual experiences of both the novice TT practitioner and the patient may differ. Hayes and Cox (1999) qualitatively assessed the similarities and differences in the TT experience from the perspective of the novice practitioner and healthy volunteers (n = 33). Like Wardell (2001), Hayes and Cox found that patients benefit from touching therapy. Patients receiving TT experienced feelings of comfort, peace, calm, and security. In addition, both the patient and the practitioner benefit from their therapeutic relationships. As both parties benefit from TT, Hayes and Cox conclude that it enhances self-awareness and facilities introspection (Hayes, 1999).

Ramnarine-Singh (1999) describes the implications of TT in preoperative patients in whom stressors (e.g., anxiety and pain) can impact the surgical outcome. Stress involves the interaction of the nervous, endocrine, and immune systems. When aroused, the nervous system triggers the release of hormones into the bloodstream, which causes the body to react (e.g., muscle tension, increased heart rate, blood pressure, and respiratory rate). Ramnarine-Singh indicates that nurses are challenged by the duty to identify stressors preoperatively to reduce patient anxiety and pain; however, TT aids nurses to overcome this challenge and implement a plan of care to reduce patient stressors. The author adds that, if data can validate the use of TT to restore balance in the energy fields of surgical patients, it can aid preoperative nurses as they attempt to control these stressors that can influence positively the patient's post-operative recovery (Ramnarine-Singh, 1999).

Reiki is a form of non-invasive healing touch by which energy is transferred to the patient via the hands of the practitioner in a particular sequence. Like all HT or TT therapies, the goal of Reiki is to restore the body's energy and balance in order to enhance the body's natural ability to heal itself. The effects of Reiki are similar to meditation in that it lowers the blood pressure, heart rate, and pulse, as well as reduces stress levels in patients. Data reported by Alandydy and Alandydy (1999) indicate that Reiki allows pre- and post-operative patients to decrease their stress levels as well as the amount of pain medication required after a procedure. The authors caution that more research needs to be conducted to verify this as well as to see if there is a correlation between the use of Reiki and the reduction in the length of hospital stay.

Le Gallez, Dimmock, and Bird (2000) describe a process, spiritual healing/therapy, much like TT or Reiki. Spiritual therapy involves the healer passing energy through the client, usually without bodily contact. In this way, the healer passes his/her hands over the client's body a few inches away without touching for approximately one to two hours weekly. Le Gallez et al. suggest that, although patients who are experiencing rheumatoid arthritis pain may not have an effect in their radiological or biochemical parameters, it can modify the patient's perception of pain. Le Gallez et al. caution that adjunct therapy such as spiritual healing should not replace conventional treatment such as drug therapy, physiotherapy, occupational therapy, and intra-articular injections for patients with rheumatoid arthritis (Le Gallez, 2000).

Assessing Spiritual Needs

As Mendyka (2000) describes culture as unique to individuals, Meravglia (1999) similarly associates personal spirituality with individualized experiences that are unique to each patient. In this way, spirituality is the experience of an individual's spirit, a connectedness to oneself and others, and an integration of human dimensions. Meravglia indicates that spirituality has been measured quantitatively in terms of spiritual well-being, spiritual perspective, self-transcendence, faith, quality of life, hope, religiousness, purpose of life, spiritual health, and spiritual coping.

Prayer, an empirical indicator of measuring spirituality, defines a connectedness with a higher power. In this way, prayer has been identified scientifically as an effective coping mechanism for ill patients. Moreover, an outcome of spirituality is the attainment of the meaning of life or motivation for life.

In this way, patients who identify their own meaning of life have benefited in both physical and emotional health as they have higher levels of self-esteem, lower levels of anxiety, distress, and social dependency, and possess an internal locus of control. Meravglia concludes that, as nurses comprehend the implications of spirituality for patient's outcomes, they are better equipped to assess the spiritual needs of their patients (Meravglia, 1999).

Prior to administering spiritually based nursing care for the infirm, nurses need to assess the spirituality of the patients. Despite the lack of tools available to identify spiritual needs of patients, tools for assessment of physiological parameters as well as psychological and sociological factors that may contribute to illness vary according to the care setting. Spiritual assessment completes the spiritual dimension of the holistic health care regimen. Although an initial spiritual assessment of the patients is instrumental in providing baseline information, their spiritual needs may change in the course of illness and treatment. Initially, a patient's spiritual assessment may be limited to asking the question regarding their religious affiliation. More extensive, standardized spiritual assessment tools include the Spiritual Perspective Scale, which measures adult spiritual perceptions; Kerrigan and Harkulich's Spiritual Assessment Tool, which identifies the spiritual needs of residents in nursing homes; and the JAREL Spiritual Well-Being Scale, which analyzes the spiritual attitudes of older adults (O'Brien, 1999).

Assessing spiritual and energy needs is imperative prior to implementing a therapeutic strategy. O'Brien (1999) discusses the assessment of spiritual needs, while Straneva (2000) focuses on assessing or scanning a patient's energy needs via the information gathering phase of TT. In this way, fluctuations in energy are evaluated via physical touch to identify areas of dissymmetry or congestion. Based on these results, practitioners attempt to transfer and restore energy in an effort to make the patient an integrated whole and promote the self-healing process. Straneva, Winstead-Fry and Kijek (1999) caution that the validity of TT as an effective therapy for ill patients is not without criticism (Straneva, 2000).

Spiritual Well-being

With respect to nursing practices, spiritual well-being integrates meaning and hope in an effort to achieve human wholeness. According to Meravglia

19

(1999), spiritual well-being is an affirmation of life in a relationship that encourages a patient's wholeness with God, self, community, and the environment. In a broader sense, general well-being refers to a personal satisfaction with life as a patient currently experiences it in the psychological and social dimensions (Meravglia, 1999). Eight characteristics of spiritual well-being are peace with God, inner peace, faith in Christ and people, good morals and health, aiding others, and being successful (O'Brien, 1999). According to Sherwood (2000), spiritual well-being is the result of healthy spirituality and serves as a foundation of holistic nursing care. In this way, spiritual well-being is an element of how one copes, solves problems, cares for oneself, and views life. Consequently, well-developed spirituality allows patients who experience healing, mutuality, and continual growth in order to achieve wholeness (Sherwood, 2000).

Nurse-Patient Relationship

In addition to the nurse's personal spirituality, factors such as the nurse's comfort level in discussing spirituality with patients, the extent of spiritual support provided in the health-care setting, and the emphasis or lack thereof on providing spiritual care to patients impact the nurse-patient relationship. General spiritual care interventions offered by nurses to patients are listed in Table 1 (O'Brien, 1999). Due to the fact that each patient has a unique spirituality, the provision of spiritual care may differ among patients.

Table 1: General Spiritual Care Interventions
—Listen to the patient regarding his/her concerns
—Provide support for the expression of patient's feelings
—Pray with the patient
—Aid patient in grieving and coping with physical and psychosocial losses
—Read favorite religious literature
—Spend time with the patient
—Offer counseling
—Offer a referral to a religious professional (e.g., chaplain)
O'Brien (1999); O'Brien (1999); Castledine (2000).

The nurse-patient relationship is critical in allowing patients to view their illnesses as a meaning-intensive experience. The nurse-client relationship is reciprocal whereby mutual spiritual growth can promote healing and well-being. As a result, both nurse and client experience satisfaction and renewal. Sherwood (2000) examined the nurse-client encounter in an effort to identify spiritual themes that influence nursing practice. Trust was one emerging theme. Nurses are trusted by patients to offer unconditional, holistic care. In addition, the mutuality of the relationship is characterized by the energy flow from nurse to client and back to the nurse as each synergistically shares his/her experience (Sherwood, 2000).

Resources for Spiritual Care

Religious and non-religious resource (Table 2) can aid the nurse in providing spiritual care to patients.

Table 2: Resources for Spiritual Care
—Pastoral care—structured and unstructured encounters
—Prayer—including:
  contemplative-meditative-intimate relationship with higher power
  ritualistic—repetition from literature or memory
  intercessory—praying on behalf of someone to a higher power
  colloquial—conversing with higher power
  petitionary—asking higher power for desired condition
  meditation
  Religious rituals
—Story-telling
—Music

Adapted from Dunn (2000), O'Brien (1999);
Wright (2000); Skokan (2000); Ameling (2000).

Pastoral Care

According to O'Brien (1999), nurses and clergy provide complementary services for the spiritual care of the
ill. Pastoral interventions are performed by religious
ministers to address the spiritual and religious needs of
others. Such interventions may be either structured (e.g.,
ceremonies, rituals) or unstructured (e.g., informal encounters). Advantages of enlisting the services of a pastoral caregiver are that he/she provides the patient with
familiar symbols and experiences and understands the
patient's religious belief system. A nurse may contact a
priest, minister, rabbi, imam, or other spiritual advisor to
inquire regarding pastoral care services (O'Brien, 1999).

Prayer

Prayer is a request or petition to a higher power to obtain a good outcome (Wright, 2000). Prayer either may be engaged in by the patient or by additional supportive people. Types of prayer are listed in Table 2. Wright cites a study in which patients receiving prayer were statistically more likely to improve their health and have fewer medical interventions and complications. In addition, Wright asserts that consciousness is the key to understanding prayer and influences one's connection with all things.

Prayer has been recognized as a spiritual treatment option in the category of mind and body control by the National Center for Complementary and Alternative Medicine (NCCAM) (Dunn, 2000). Ameling (2000) cites a recent *Time*/CNN poll which found that 82 percent of Americans believe that prayer can cure serious health conditions, 73 percent indicate that praying for others can cure health problems, and 64 percent want their doctors to pray with them (Dunn, 2000; Barnes, 2000). Dunn and Horgas (2000) categorize prayer as a spiritual cognitive therapy used by elders, in particular, to reappraise and reevaluate stressful life events, diminish the negative effects of stress, and maintain optimum levels of health. In order to play an instrumental role in the healing and coping strategies of older adults, nurses must recognize the importance of prayer as a spiritual self-care modality (Dunn, 2000).

Dunn and Horgas (2000) add that prayer is the most universally recognized religious practice by which individuals commune with a deity or Creator. A Gallup poll survey indicates that while 90 percent of Americans pray, the prevalence of prayer increases with age as 73 percent praying at least once daily. Dunn and Horgas cite research that indicates that older adults are more apt to practice prayer as a coping strategy because they possess a greater ability to integrate cognitive and emotional processes and use prayer as a passive, interpersonal, and emotion-focused coping process.

Older people are at a high risk for stress due to deteriorating health, chronic illness, pain, and multiple losses (e.g., from death of relations). In addition, Dunn and Horgas summarize an extensive body of literature indicating that both positive physical and psychological outcomes were found in participants who prayed and who suspected others praying for them (Dunn, 2000).

Based on previous reports, Dunn and Horgas (2000) designed a pilot study that investigated prayer as a spiritual treatment modality and coping strategy in elderly individuals (n = 50) from various religious and demographic (e.g., ethnicity, marital status, educational status) backgrounds. Information was gathered via questionnaires and interviews. Dunn and Horgas found that the diverse community-dwelling elders enlisted prayer to cope with stress in their lives.

In particular, women and Blacks reported using prayer more often to cope as compared to men and Whites. Data also failed to show differences in prayer use in married, single, divorced, widowed, Catholic, or Protestant individuals. Dunn and Horgas's findings are consistent with those previously reported. Moreover, the participants in the study reported prayer as the most frequently used alternative treatment. Participants who used prayer were more likely to be optimistic and self-reliant in their coping strategies; thus, it is instrumental in maintaining health and well-being (Dunn, 2000).

Although Dunn and Horgas (2000) and Wright (2000) espouse the benefits of prayer on the coping strategies and overall health of patients, Ameling (2000) cautions that these assertions are met with some skepticism. For lack of tangible evidence, a portion of the medical community views prayer as a harmless modality, certainly not intrinsic to healing. Regardless, Ameling views prayer as an ancient healing practice not widely available in our current health-care system.

As an endorsement for the use of prayer, specifically meditation, in the health-care setting, Ameling cites data that suggest that meditation lowers respiratory rates, heart rates, blood pressure, and skin temperature as well as producing a sense of calm and well-being. As the health-care system shows renewed interest in the healing power of prayer without sacrificing critical judgment, spirituality and prayer practices may become integrated into holistic nursing practice (Ameling, 2000).

Religious Rituals

Providing support for religious rituals proven meaningful to an ailing patient should be an integral part of a nurse's spiritual care regimen. Religious rituals are groups of behaviors that mirror and honor religious or spiritual beliefs. For example, a nurse may provide a prayer rug for a Muslim patient who is devoted to pray formally five times daily (e.g., the five pillars of Islam) facing the east (Mecca). O'Brien (1999) indicates that religious rituals have a profoundly healing power for patients, especially those who are acutely ill.

Storytelling

Storytelling has proven to be a valuable tool to aid patients in coping with chronic illness. Storytelling serves as a mechanism by which the patient organizes his or her personal experience and thought in order to enable him/her to reflect on and make sense of life. By sharing personal experiences with others, patients often experience a sense of connectedness and intimacy that is related to spirituality. As a result, spiritual caregivers can facilitate the healing process by allowing the patient to engage in storytelling and ask interested questions to encourage the patient to converse (Skokan, 2000).

Music

Music thanatology is considered a palliative medical therapy that is concerned both with the alleviation of physiological pain and spiritual and interior distress. Music thanatology is rooted in monastic medicine that was practiced in the Middle Ages. Monks associated with a Benedictine monastery in France during the late eleventh century adopted a twofold medical program based on the care of both the body and soul. As a result, the story of the Benedictine monastery served as a historical inspiration for music thanatology, now in its twenty-eighth year. Horrigan (2001) adds that, in order to deliver prescriptive music, one needs polyphonic instrument, such as the piano, organ, flute, guitar, or harp.

In effect, the music emanating from the instruments bathes the patient in sound, which accumulates over the entire body in an effort to promote the introspection of the patient. Consequently, the music is a non-talk modality, which promotes spirituality without preaching or dogma (Horrigan, 2001).

Horrigan (2001) suggests that the effects of music can be measured via physiological, quantitative parameters such as the pulse and respiratory patterns, body temperature, countenance, gesture, skin color, etc., pre-, mid-, and post-session. For example, a sign of internal peace would be manifested as the pulse and heart beat change, tremors subside or lessen, and facial grimaces soften. The musician accomplishes this by synchronizing the music with the heartbeat and pulse of the patient in order to accompany the patient physiologically. Conversely, some effects (e.g., the achievement of internal peace and introspection) in the patient's state of being cannot be measured (Horrigan, 2001).

Parish Nursing

Due to the emphasis of healing and wholeness in the faith practices of many religions, churches have a lengthy history of involvement in healing and providing health care. Consequently, healing was an essential part of the early Christian church's ministry. Religious hospitals and monastic orders were established to care for the sick and infirm during that time. The church's interest in the role of faith as it relates to physical, emotional, and spiritual damage was revived in the nineteenth century (Brendtro, 2000).

Beginning in the mid-1980s, parish nursing was initiated as a specialty practice to promote the health of the faith community by integrating theological, sociological, and physiological perspectives of health and healing into religious services. In 2000, an estimated 2,500 nurses worked in the parish nursing system as a result of the rising interest in the link between spirituality and health (Metzger, 2000). Whisnant (1999) adds that parish nursing is growing and will serve a dominant role in the future of nursing.

Parish nurses are registered nurses who facilitate holistic health for a faith community. Sometimes, a church employs a parish nurse to function as a member of the ministerial team to provide nursing services to parishioners. In addition, a hospital or other health-care institution may enlist the services of a parish nurse in partnership with a local parish as a way of integrating health promotion into a particular community. Four types of parish nurses are: congregation-based volunteer, congregation-based paid, institution-based volunteer, and institution-based paid.

O'Brien (1999) confirms that parish nurses function as organizers, educators, and liaisons with the health-care community in an effort to encourage a relationship between one's faith and health. In this way, parish nurses view health as including an individual's physical, emotional, social, and spiritual being (Brendtro, 2000).

Parish nursing ministries are emerging throughout the United States. In particular, DeSchepper (1999) describes a system-wide effort by Avera Health Facilities to develop parish nursing in the Midwest. In order to get the system established, parish leaders and members, as well as local healthcare providers, needed to be educated regarding the mission of the ministry as well as the services provided to the community. Avera formed partnerships with educational facilities in order to provide continuing health education for parish nurses and nursing students.

Avera leaders consider spiritual support for the parish nurses, themselves, a priority; therefore, they periodically offer a retreat for parish nurses and those who support them where they can seek counsel in order to replenish their spirits. Regarding the benefits of parish nursing, DeSchepper suggests that the communication and education skills of the parish nurse raise the awareness of church staff, offering them a redefined sense of calling and ministry to the whole person and the community (DeSchepper, 1999).

Similarly, Metzger (2000) elaborates on DeSchepper's (1999) assertions and details the role of the parish nurse and the skills needed to perform their job. Parish nursing is considered to be health promotion within the context of a faith community's values, beliefs, and practices. In effect, parish nurses are a vital link between members of a congregation and physicians, dentists, hospitals, managed-care programs, and allied health-care organizations.

Although some are paid, Metzger indicates that the majority of parish nurses are part-time volunteers. Regarding the responsibilities of parish nurses, they are not able to provide direct clinical care or administer medications. Rather, they are equipped to conduct a needs assessment for patients and schedule introductory activities such as blood-pressure screenings. In addition to applying their exceptional skills for needs assessment, parish nurses promote health education via counseling community members, teaching and organizing volunteers, planning community outreach programs, and directing members to appropriate health and social services. Metzger concludes that parish nurses positively influence the health of community members, while reducing the costs of health care and improving their quality of life (Metzger, 2000).

Brendtro and Leuning (2000) concur with Metzger's (2000) assertion that church-based health programs, such as parish nursing, are cost-effective. In this way, a church-based program attempts to teach members of the faith community regarding what constitutes a healthy life-style from a holistic perspective consistent with their faith, morals, and values. In this way, educated people have the advantage and encouragement to live healthy life-styles and, therefore, may avoid expensive health-care costs. In addition, churches often have existing educational programs and committees already familiar with parishioners that serve as potential avenues for the delivery of health programs. In comparison, if these systems were not in place, revenue and personnel would be required to implement the services; therefore, having these resources already available through the church is cost-effective (Brendtro, 2000).

Faith community nursing (FCN) is synonymous with parish nursing to the extent that nurses work out of a faith community (e.g., churches, church-based school, aged-care facility, or community agency). FCNs are volunteer or paid registered nurses who practice on individuals within the faith community first, then the geographic or cultural group surrounding the community. FCNs offer health promotion and disease prevention activities, as well as education and counseling to people and small groups.

Issues addressed by FCNs include, but are not limited to, managing a crying baby, grief and loss, bereavement, coping with teenagers, and dealing with dementia. In addition, FCNs are client advocates who aid people in navigating the health system while locating appropriate government, community, church, or family resources to direct their health issues. With respect to the chronically ill, FCNs manage their care by incorporating dimensions, such as mind, body, and spirit, of the whole individual and their significant relationships (Anonymous, 1999).

Acutely and Chronically Ill Patients

Depending on factors such as age, religious tradition, and the gravity of their condition, adult patients suffering from acute illness have diverse spiritual needs. In fact, the spiritual beliefs of patients may become increasingly important as they become acutely ill. O'Brien (1999) and O'Brien (1999) indicate that the spiritual health of acutely and chronically ill patients is an essential factor in aiding them in their coping strategy. In fact, O'Brien cites reports suggesting that a significant correlation exists between spiritual health and a patient's general evaluation of his or her overall physical health. In this way, spiritual health is the state of well-being or interior state of peace and joy, free from abnormal anxiety, guilt, or feeling of sinfulness (O'Brien, 1999).

Skokan and Bader (2000) assessed the influence of spirituality and spiritual experiences on the health and well-being of chronically ill patients (n = 162), many of whom had life-threatening illnesses. In analyzing data from questionnaires, Skokan and Bader identified lessons or themes. First, the chronically ill patients needs to engage in discovering the meaning of life. Spiritual caregivers facilitate this by aiding the patient in identifying what he/she has lost as a result of the chronic illness and the new meaning of their limitations. Caregivers have an ability to validate whatever the patient deems meaningful and are aware of the patient's values, concerns, and beliefs.

Moreover, Skokan and Bader found that a patient's religious upbringing influences the ways in which he/she copes with his/her illness. Furthermore, spiritual caregivers help patients reach a point of acceptance and peace by respecting their spiritual and cultural diversity, aiding them to accept what is life-giving about their religious heritage and achieve closure (Skokan, 2000).

Spiritual Healing and Patients with Anxiety Disorders

Aside from patients who are acutely and chronically ill as well as candidates for surgery, patients with anxiety disorders use alternative therapies such as spiritual healing. Kessler, Soukup, Davis, and Foster et al. (2001) assessed the use of alternative therapies in patients experiencing anxiety attacks in addition to severe depression. Kessler et al. assert that use of these alternative therapies will most likely increase as insurance coverage expands. Finally, health care professionals who inquire regarding a patient's use of an alternative therapy (e.g., relaxation, spirituality) ultimately may maximize the usefulness and efficacy of the therapy (Kessler, 2001).

Emotional Needs of Atheists

Atheists deny the existence of God and propose a significant challenge to nurses who attempt to minister to their emotional needs. Although atheists do not share the religious beliefs of others, O'Brien (1999) suggests that they do, of course, have emotional needs. It is the responsibility of the nurse to recognize this and be creative and compassionate in their assessment and interventions. Skokan and Bader (2000) add that spirituality is expressed in many ways other than through religious activities; rather experiencing relationships among music, art, and pets can provide spiritual experiences for patients.

Conclusion

With the advent of the holistic health movement, spiritual care of the ill has become a legitimately recognized activity within the domain of nursing (O'Brien, 1999; Anonymous, 2000). As a result, nursing textbooks offer advice that assesses a patient's spiritual needs as well as providing spiritual care are essential components of the nursing profession. For parish nurses, in particular, healing and holistic care are at the core of their services. By taking a holistic health-care approach, individuals are encouraged to make healthy life-style choices, which ultimately improve the quality of their lives (Bowman, 1999).

In gaining a historical perspective of the caring, commitment, and spirituality of pre-Christian and Christian forefathers, contemporary nurses internalize new meaning as they minister to the ill. Although the spiritual care provided by nurses is unrecognized and rarely documented in the patients' charts, it is nonetheless an important part of practice (O'Brien, 1999). In recent years, the majority of health-care providers, whether religious or secular, have focused increased attention on the role of spirituality in healing (Skokan, 2000).

Neglecting the spiritual dimension of care may have detrimental effects on the patient's condition (O'Brien, 1999). Spiritual needs include the desire for support, compassion, knowledgeable caring, forgiveness, love, hope, and trust. Unmet spiritual needs cause patients to feel alienated, lonely, isolated, as well as impair healing and satisfaction with life circumstances (Sherwood, 2000).

Skokan and Bader (2000) assert that spirituality provides patients with hope, strength, and emotional support they may need in order to gain a peaceful satisfaction as they come to terms with their illness. In fact, Skokan and Bader add that some studies describe a connection between spiritual well-being and physical cure. In this way, cure refers to the physical alleviation of the signs and symptoms of disease at the anatomical level (Skokan, 2000). Sherwood (2000) adds that the nature of the nurse-client interaction impacts outcomes.

In order for the relationship to have a positive impact, it must be founded on honesty, flexibility, advocacy, and support as nurses offer patients interventions that focus on maintaining a connection and integrating the use of self (Sherwood, 2000). In addition, knowledge of spirituality can be applied to nursing assessments to promote positive patient outcomes (Cavendish, 2000). Meravglia (1999) adds that spiritual, psychological, and physical well-being are outcomes of spirituality.

Nurses encourage a positive attitude and attributes in a patient's life via an abundance of spiritual care interventions. Parish nurses, in particular, serve as a valuable resource to empower community members to make decisions concerning their health (Brendtro, 2000). Holistic or energy-based therapies, such as HT, address the spiritual needs of both the client and the practitioner. Similarly, Straneva (2000) asserts that TT promotes the exchange of energy from the practitioner to the patient in an effort to restore the patient's energy field, self-healing,

34

and well-being, enhancing their overall quality of life. Wardell (2001) asserts that, in order for the nursing profession to enter and remain in the forefront of holistic health-care, spiritual issues must be addressed and developed via alternative interventions such as HT. Undoubtedly, spiritual nursing care is essential for professional nurses; however nurses often are uncomfortable with this aspect of care. Emblen and Pesut (2001) offer reasons for this discomfort, which include an inadequate education, anxiety regarding the discussion of spiritual matters, confusion about the definition of spirituality, and the assumed incompatibility between spirituality and the scientific model of nursing. Dossey (2000) argues that science, a long-time enemy of spirituality, is considering that the condition of the soul and spirit are essential to health. Nonetheless, these barriers to the implementation of spirituality in nursing can be accomplished through the design of new models to assist nurses in offering patients spiritual care.

Finally, addressing issues such as holism and spirituality in nursing may create a frame of reference wherein nursing educators can adapt curricula and classroom or job experiences to encourage nurses to assist patients in self-care. Nurses who are educated regarding the implications of their own spirituality are better equipped to heal via the creation of harmony, congruity, and integration. Other than providing continuing education for nurses in issues of spirituality and healing, organizational culture can encourage the spiritual development of both the client and the caregiver.

As the healthcare system attempts to offer patients a feasible adjunct to their traditional medical regimens, organizations need to display readiness to take on this challenge, develop an educational plan, and attempt to integrate alternative therapies into existing programs. An effective educational plan may include both course work as well as the acquisition of practical skills via an apprenticeship (Mullane, 2000).

As members of an organization share a common vision of spiritual health care, they are progressing toward reaching a culture of healing. In this way, an organization that has a strong, ongoing effort to encourage conscious spiritual health-care behaviors in its employees is more likely to possess a thriving healing culture in which the mission and values of a particular health ministry will flourish (Agnew, 1999).

In making this transition from strictly traditional to incorporating alternative practices, the nurses' role will expand to encompass the spiritual as well as the physical and psychological care of patients.

Three
Implications, Recommendations, and Conclusions

Implications

Consideration of a patient's spiritual needs is becoming paramount when designing therapeutic strategies for patient care. As a result, services provided by nurses proceed from the traditional, medical services to the spiritually based through the implementation of alternative or complementary care. This holistic approach of integrating services for the mind, body, and spirit has proven to be effective in healing the infirm.

Consequently, failing to consider a patient's spirituality when administering care may have negative consequences for the patient (O'Brien, 1999). Spiritual needs of individuals include, but are not limited to, the desire for support, compassion, knowledgeable care, forgiveness, love, hope, and trust. Moreover, spirituality offers patients the support they desire to gain—peaceful satisfaction as they come to terms with their illness. If the patient's spiritual needs remain unaddressed and, therefore, unmet, patients experience loneliness, alienation, and isolation, which may hinder healing and personal satisfaction (Sherwood, 2000).

The nurse-client relationship is instrumental in the

promotion of positive patient outcomes. In this way, nurses provide patients with interventions that focus on maintaining a connection with a higher power as well as integrating the use of self in order to empower the patient and promote self-care. Spiritual resources include touch- or energy-based therapies (e.g., healing touch, therapeutic touch, and Reiki), prayer, storytelling, music, and pastoral care/religious rituals.

Spiritually based therapies have a positive effect on patient outcomes. Straneva (2000) believes that therapies such as these allow the exchange of energy from the practitioner to the patient in an effort to restore the patient's energy field, self-healing, and well-being, resulting in a enhancement of their general quality of life. Although they may not cure the patient of the illness, spiritually based therapies have a healing effect on the patient and bring them the inner peace they need to come to terms and cope with their situation.

Undoubtedly, the historical perspective of spirituality in nursing presented in this thesis suggests that spirituality has proven to be an essential factor to consider when ministering to an ill patient. Throughout the ages, religious rituals, praying, and storytelling, as examples, were ways in which individuals dealt with illness, whether it be their own or someone else's.

The functions of caregivers and nurses have evolved from the mysticism of pre-Christian societies in which gifts were offered to the gods in return for a favorable outcome to those of specific religious orders of nurses focusing on meeting the physical as well as the spiritual needs of patients in an effort to imitate Jesus Christ.

Recommendations

Despite the consistent medical advances occurring throughout history, spiritual interventions have remained constant. What has proven to be effective in retrospect still remains effective today in terms of addressing the spiritual needs of patients. While spirituality is deep-rooted in nursing history, somewhere along the line, the profession moved away from spiritually based therapies.

Perhaps this is due to the skepticism of the medical community. As nurses enter into the forefront of holistic health care, they need to have a model from which to draw upon in order to provide patients with the spiritually based alternative therapies they need. By gaining historical perspective, nurses are educated and receive adequate support in order to design the ways to provide patients with effective holistic services that result in enhancing positive patient outcomes. The holistic services may include spiritually based interventions proven to be effective throughout the ages.

Conclusions

As a renewed interest in holistic health care via alternative and complementary therapies emerges, there is an increasing demand on nurses to integrate spiritual care into services they provide to patients. Consequently, nurses are challenged with assessing and meeting not only the physical, but also the spiritual needs of patients. In addition, nurses are at a disadvantage in this role change because they are faced with a paradigm shift from traditional alternative practices, and they are not properly educated or supported in doing so.

Nurses may be educated via many sources. Continuing or classroom education is beginning to address issues of spirituality and healing with respect to the provision of nursing services. Internships also provide the hands-on experience that nurses may need effectively to integrate spirituality into their regimen. In addition to internships, a historical perspective of spirituality and nursing serves as a model for nurses to refer to when attempting to meet the spiritual needs of their patients. Insight into what spiritually based practices are effective in enhancing patient outcomes gives nurses a raving endorsement and insight into which strategies they should model. Furthermore, ancient remedies are validated constantly as positive patient outcomes are documented throughout the ages.

Whether or not nurses are equipped and educated is one issue that can be addressed and remedied through continuing education, training, and research; however, whether or not nursing are comfortable with offering spiritually based therapies to patients is another issue. Perhaps with education and training comes a particular comfort level adequate for a nurse to accept his/her new role and responsibilities.

Nonetheless, nurses who are comfortable with their own spirituality have proven to be better adept at addressing the spiritual needs of others. Nurses who are uncomfortable with addressing such needs should recognize this shortcoming and refer the patient to the appropriate services as opposed to relinquishing responsibility and allowing the patient's spiritual needs to remain unmet.

Lastly, although evidence does exist to support the use of spiritually based therapies in an effort to promote patient healing, it is met with some skepticism in the scientific community. Whether or not these therapies produce a placebo effect is unclear. For example, if a patient deeply believes that an intervention is going to have a positive effect on his/her health status, he/she subconsciously can alter his/her physiology in order to achieve this goal. Therefore, it is not the intervention directly that is having the effect; rather, it is the patient's perception of the desired effects of the intervention.

Nonetheless, these spiritually based interventions have proven throughout history to be beneficial to patients. Placebo effect or not, the bottom line is that patients are exhibiting self-healing and empowerment, thus enhancing their overall quality of life. Nurses, whether they believe in these spiritually based therapies or not, are charged with the responsibility of providing them to patients as their roles shift from being traditional to holistic caregivers.

References

Agnew, M. (1999). "The spiritual side of illness." *Health Progress.* 80 (4), 66.

Alandydy, P.; Alandydy, K. (1999). "Using Reiki to support surgical patients." *Journal of Nursing Care.* 13 (4), 89–91.

Ameling, A. (2000). "Prayer: An ancient healing practice becomes new again." *Holistic Nursing Practice.* 14 (3), 40–48.

Anonymous. (1999). "Faith community nursing: Holistic care for communities." *Australian Nursing Journal.* 6 (10, 31).

Anonymous. (2000). *Nursing Standard.* "Spirituality in nursing practice." 15 (11), 29.

Barnes, L., Plotnikoff, G., Fox, K., Pendleton, S. (2000). "Spirituality, religion, and pediatrics: Intersecting worlds of healing." *Pediatrics.* 106 (4), 899–908.

Bowman, C.; Schultz, M. (1999). "Four keys to success in parish nursing." *Health Progress.* 80 (2), 40.

Brendtro, M.; Leuning, C. (2000). "Nurses in churches: A population-focused clinical option." *Journal of Nursing Education.* 39 (6), 285.

Castledine G. (2000). "Spirituality and being a 'friend of the patient.' " *British Journal of Nursing.* 9 (1), 62.

Cavendish, R., Luise, B., Horne, K., Bauer, M., et al. (2000). "Opportunities for enhanced spirituality relevant to well adults." *Nursing Diagnosis.* 11 (4), 151–163.

DeSchepper, C. (1999). "Healthier communities through parish nursing. *Health Progress.* 80 (4), 56.

Dossey, B. (2000). "Spirituality and nursing: Florence Nightingale's legacy for the nurse as an instrument of healing." *Dean's Notes (National Student Nurses Association).* 21 (5), 1.

Dunn, K; Horgas, A. (2000). "The prevalence of prayer as a spiritual self-care modality in elders." *Journal of Holistic Nursing.* 18 (4), 337–351.

Emblen, J; Pesut B. (2001). "Strengthening transcendent meaning: A model for spiritual nursing care of patients experiencing suffering." *Journal of Holistic Nursing.* 19 (1), 42˙56.

Hayes, J; Cox, C. (1999). "The experience of therapeutic touch from a nursing perspective." *British Journal of Nursing.* 8 (18), 1249.

Holstein, M. (2000). "A spiritual role for the elderly." *Health Progress.* 81 (2), 12.

Horrigan, B. (2001). "Therese Schroeder-Shekere music thanatology and spiritual care for the dying." *Alternative Therapies in Health and Medicine.* 7 (1), 68.

Kessler, R., Soukup, J., Davis, R., Foster, D., et al. (2001). "The use of complementary and alternative therapies to treat anxiety and depression in the United States." *American Journal of Psychiatry.* 158 (2), 289–294.

Koehn, M. (2000). "Alternative and complementary therapies for labor and birth: An application of Kolcaba's theory of holistic comfort." *Holistic Nursing Practice.* 15 (1), 66–77.

Le Gallez, P., Dimmock, S.; Bird H. (2000). "Spiritual healing as adjunct therapy for rheumatoid arthritis." *British Journal Holistic Nursing.* 9 (11), 695.

Marshall, ES; Wall, BM. (1999). "Religion, gender, and autonomy: A comparison of two religious women's groups in nursing and hospitals in the late nineteenth and early twentieth centuries." *Advances in Nursing Science.* 22 (1), 22.

Mendkya, B. (2000). "Exploring the culture of nursing: A theory-driven practice." *Holistic Nursing Practice.* 15 (1), 32–41.

Meravglia, M. (1999). "Critical analysis of spirituality and its empirical indicators." *Journal of Holistic Nursing.* 17 (1), 18–33.

Metzger, S. (2000). "Parish nursing: Integrating body, mind, and spirit." *Nursing.* 30 (12), HH6.

Mullane, M. (2000). "A glance back in time." *Nursing Forum.* 35 (4), 41–45.

O'Brien, M. (1999). "A spiritual history of nursing." In: O'Brien, M.Ed. *Spirituality in Nursing: Standing on Holy Ground.* Jones and Bartlett: Boston. 1–17, 21–52, 56–81, 85–116, 118–142, 1438–170, 174–202.

O'Callaghan, J. (2001). "Do rituals rule over research evidence?" *Australian Nursing Journal.* 8 (8), 39.

Ramnarine-Singh, S. (1999). "The surgical significance of therapeutic touch." *AORN Journal.* 69 (2), 358–369.

Sherwood, G. (2000). "The power of nurse-client encounters: Interpreting spiritual themes." *Journal of Holistic Nursing.* 18 (2), 159–175.

Skokan, L., Bader, D. (2000). "Spirituality and healing." *Health Progress.* 81 (1), 38.

Slater, V., Maloney, J., Krau, S., Eckert, C. (1999). "Journey to holism." *Journal of Holistic Nursing.* 17 (4), 365–383.

Straneva, J. (2000). "Therapeutic touch coming of age." *Holistic Nursing Practice.* 14 (3), 1–13.

Wardell, D. (2001). "Spirituality of healing touch participants." *Journal of Holistic Nursing.* 19 (1), 71–86.

Whisnant S. (1999). "The parish nurse: Tending to the spiritual side of health." *Holistic Nursing Practice.* 14 (1), 84–86.

Winstead-Fry, P., Kijek, J. (1999). "An integrative review and meta-analysis of therapeutic touch research." *Alternative Therapies in Health and Medicine.* 5 (6), 58.

Wong, T., Pang, M. (2000). "Holism and caring: Nursing

in the Chinese health care culture." *Holistic Nursing Practice.* 15 (1), 12–21.

Wright S. (2000). "Praying for good health." *Nursing Standard.* 15 (2), 27.